Prof. Mehdia GANDI
Prof. Zitouni BENABDELGHANI
Prof. Mohamed AMARI

How to update my knowledge of topical Bionanocomposites

Prof. Mehdia GANDI
Prof. Zitouni BENABDELGHANI
Prof. Mohamed AMARI

How to update my knowledge of topical Bionanocomposites

Book for pharmaceutical engineering students

ScienciaScripts

Imprint

Any brand names and product names mentioned in this book are subject to trademark, brand or patent protection and are trademarks or registered trademarks of their respective holders. The use of brand names, product names, common names, trade names, product descriptions etc. even without a particular marking in this work is in no way to be construed to mean that such names may be regarded as unrestricted in respect of trademark and brand protection legislation and could thus be used by anyone.

Cover image: www.ingimage.com

This book is a translation from the original published under ISBN 978-620-6-71218-3.

Publisher:
Sciencia Scripts
is a trademark of
Dodo Books Indian Ocean Ltd. and OmniScriptum S.R.L publishing group

120 High Road, East Finchley, London, N2 9ED, United Kingdom
Str. Armeneasca 28/1, office 1, Chisinau MD-2012, Republic of Moldova, Europe
Printed at: see last page
ISBN: 978-620-7-63654-9

How to update my knowledge of topical Bionanocomposites

By: *Professor Mehdia GANDI.*

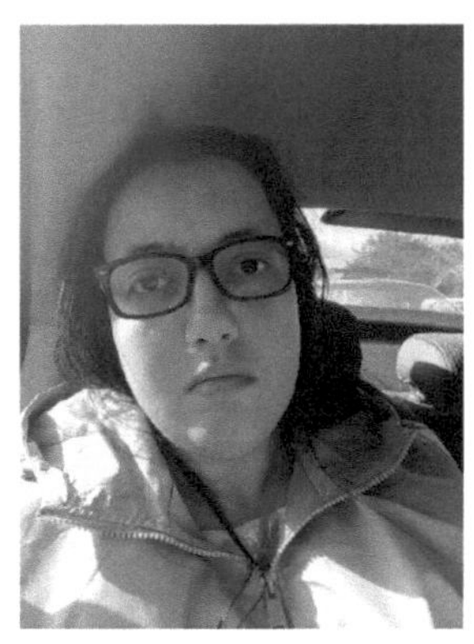

Temporary researcher at USTHB, in the Faculty of Mechanical and Process Engineering & the Faculty of Chemistry, working on pharmaceutical technologies.

Signing sessions

This book is dedicated to my parents and my small, or large, family, as well as to all my teachers, in particular.

Contents

Film Dressings :

Given its easy availability, relatively inexpensive price and environmental friendliness, beaver oil was used in a 2015 study as a matrix for wound-healing film dressings filled with modified CS-ZnO NPs (by adding NaOH and sonication). Among the analyses carried out on the dressings are their :

- Morphology (roughness...in short, for marketing purposes).

- Structure (to guarantee a better therapist effect).

- Thermal stability (for safe storage at outside temperatures).

- Hydrophilia (absorbing wound exudates).

- Biodegradability (to protect the environment).

- Cytocompatibility (minimal cytotoxicity).

- Barrier properties (watertightness of dressings).

- Viscoelastic properties (dressings that attach well and don't tear easily).

- Anti-bacterial properties.

When the concentration of CS-ZnO nanofillers NPs increases ↑ in a biopansement matrix and plasticized by freeze-drying (sous-vide):

- Hydrophilia increases ↑ (drying of wound exudates).

- Increased thermal stability ↑ (guaranteed preservation) .

- Increased porosity ↑ (better wound drying).

- Water vapor transmission rate (WVTR) increases ↑ (better wound hydration).

- Oxygen permeability increases ↑ (a well-ventilated wound) (Díez-Pascual; 2015).

References :

Díez-Pascual, A.M.; Díez-Vicente, A.L., (2015). Wound Healing Bionanocomposites Based on Castor Oil Polymeric Films Reinforced with Chitosan-Modified ZnO Nanoparticles, Biomac, 16, 2631-2644.

Recent advances in the nano-engineering of cellulose as a carrier of active ingredients or incorporated into medical devices.

Over the last decade, there has been a growing demand for the substitution of synthetic materials with platforms of natural origin, to minimize their undesirable footprints on biomedicine, the environment and ecosystems. Among natural materials, cellulose, the world's most abundant biopolymer with key properties such as biocompatibility, bio-renewability and durability, has received considerable attention. The hierarchical structure of cellulose fibers, the main constituents of the plant cell wall, has been nanoengineered and fused into biomedical block constructs, providing nanoscale infrastructure within pharmaceutical sub-works or devices, such as implants and surgical instruments, in nanomedicine. Microorganisms, such as certain types of bacteria, are another source of nanocelluloses known as nanocellulose bacteria (NCB), which benefit from high purity and crystallinity. Chemical and mechanical treatments of cellulose fibrils, made up of alternating crystalline and amorphous regions, produce cellulose nanocrystals (CNC), hairy cellulose nanocrystals (Hairy CNC) and cellulose nanofibrils (CNF), with dimensions ranging from a few nanometers to several microns. Cellulose nanocrystals and nanofibrils can easily bind to drugs, proteins and nanoparticles via physical interactions, or be chemically modified to covalently accommodate cargoes. Surface engineering properties, such as chemical functionality, charge, surface area, crystallinity and hydrophilicity, play a central role in controlling cargo loading/rejection capacity and rate, stability, toxicity, immunogenicity and biodegradation of nanocellulose-based delivery platforms. This review provides an overview of recent advances in the nano-engineering of cellulose crystals and fibrils to develop vehicles, encompassing colloidal nanoparticles, hydrogels, aerogels, films, coatings, capsules and membranes, for the delivery of a wide range of bioactive cargoes, such as chemotherapy (anti-cancer) drugs, anti-inflammatory agents, antibacterial and probiotic compounds (antibiotics of bacterial or yeast origin, in short made from microorganisms naturally present in the human body, useful as antidiarrheals, and to treat certain infections) (Sheikhi ; 2018) .

Mots-Clés Du Manuscrit (Sheikhi; 2018) :

Nanocellulose; Cellulose nanocrystals; Hairy nanocellulose; Bacterial cellulose; Cellulose nanofibrils; Drug delivery; Wound healing; Cancer treatment.

References :

Amir Sheikhi, Joel Hayashi, James Eichenbaum, Mark Gutin, Nicole Kuntjoro, Danial Khorsandi, Ali Khademhosseini, Recent advances in nanoengineering cellulose for cargo delivery. Corel (2018), https://doi.org/10.1016/j.jconrel.2018.11.024.

The Application of Biopolymer Hydrogel Products in Tissue Engineering

Decades have passed since the concept of tissue engineering was first put forward, and in recent years it has developed rapidly. Tissue substitutes, for artificial blood vessels, skin, bone and heart repair, have been widely studied not only in the research field, but also in clinical cases. For tissue engineering, scaffolds, also known as structural composites or block composites, are an indispensable component, which have also seen a shift from synthetic to natural materials with good biocompatibility. On the other hand, hydrogels prepared from natural polymers have properties similar to those of the ecosystem environment, and have the advantage of promoting cell adhesion, proliferation and targeting. These medical bionanocomposites, in their various forms, thanks to their biocompatibility, biodegradability and porosity, are commonly applied in cell culture neurogenesis, cardiac repair (pacemaker or = pacemaker or = cardiac battery) and bone and cartilage reconstruction (prostheses). Although a great deal of research has been carried out into tissue-engineered scaffolds, few have been commercialized, even after overcoming the drawback of insufficient mechanical properties. Since the human body is delicate, balancing the strength of scaffolds with the rate of tissue formation is one of the most difficult problems to solve, limiting their uses in the present. In addition, ensuring blood and tissue biocompatibility, to overcome rejection by the immune system, also requires a large number of clinical experiments.

With the advent of three-dimensional printing technology, and artificial intelligence, the manufacture of bio-hydrogels, would be more practical and intelligent, and could overcome the problems of existing medical devices, such as implants and prostheses...and this would benefit a greater number of patients, with organ damage (Yang; 2020).

References :

Yang, J.; Sun, X.; Zhang, Y.; Chen, Y.; (2020). The application of natural polymer based hydrogels in tissue engineering. Hydrogels Based on Natural Polymers, Chapter 10 (273-307).

New Asymmetric Chitosan-Polyvinylpyrrolidone-Nanocellulose Dressings "CS-PVP-NC Systems": In Vitro and In Vivo Evaluation :

A wound can be defined as an acute injury, which damages the dermis of the skin and disrupts the normal anatomical (body) relationship of tissues due to an accident or suture. Wound healing is a multifactorial, physiological and complicated process, and generally needs to be covered by a dressing immediately after damage, as complications associated with wounds include infection, deformity, scar tissue proliferation and bleeding. Several dressing products are commercially available in the form of: non-adherent dressings, emollient dressings, film dressings, hydrocolloids, hydrogels, hydrofibers, foam dressings, antimicrobial dressings, charcoal dressings and composite dressings. In recent years, wound healing based on biopolymer dressings has been widely used, such as the abundant natural chitosan, due to its non-toxic character, and its biocompatible, biodegradable, moisturizing properties. What's more, it's readily available.

Chitosan has all the ideal properties for accelerating the wound-healing process. Chitosan is a β-1,4-bonded polymer of glucosamine (2-amino-2-deoxy-β-D-glucose) and smaller amounts of N-acetyl glucosamine. It is derived from chitin (poly-N-acetyl glucosamine), the second most abundant biopolymer after cellulose. Chitosan is a unique natural polymer with properties such as biocompatibility and biodegradability, all of which derive from the presence of the primary amine group on the backbone of its structure. It can be used in the treatment of wounds and burns due to its intrinsic antimicrobial property and hemostatic potential. A great deal of research in this field concludes that chitosan remains a suitable treatment for wounds and burns.

However, the application of chitosan can be limited by its poor mechanical properties, and the loss of its structural integrity. To overcome these drawbacks, chitosan is blended with synthetic polymers to broaden its range of applications. Biopolymer blending, too, is one of the most effective methods of creating new biomaterials with the desired properties. Chitosan/PVP blends have been attracting interest over the past decade, as their properties can be tailored to suit desirable needs and applications.

Polyvinylpyrrolidone (PVP), also known as polyvidone or povidone, is a synthetic, water-soluble, biocompatible polymer used for many biomedical applications, including wound dressings, and represents the main component in the development of temporary skin coverings, due to its transparency. PVP combines with iodine to form an antiseptic povidone-iodine solution with excellent disinfectant properties that are used for many medical purposes. However, skin disinfection with povidone-iodine is less common than for disinfecting surgical instruments, due to its undesirable effects on the skin, such as the risk of irritability, burns and severe allergic reactions in some patients. Several studies have reported the compatibility of chitosan and PVP, as they are easily miscible with each other.

The introduction of nanotechnology is one of the most important recent advances.

In this field, effective modification of blends is achieved to improve the properties of biopolymers, thus broadening their fields of application. Nanocellulose (NC) is a cellulose derivative composed of a network of nano-sized fibers, which has attracted a great deal of attention and interest in recent decades, due to its value-added biomedical applications. In recent years, considerable attention has been paid to nanocellulose-based materials, and their applications in wound dressing. Nanocellulose is suitable for wound dressing applications, as it possesses a number of interesting features, including its fine structure, high specific surface area, good mechanical and rheological properties, barrier properties, lack of toxicity and biocompatibility. Recently, several studies have investigated the potential of ternary polymer blends in biomedical applications.

Today, many polymers, including natural materials, synthetic materials and combinations of both, are combined with nanoparticles to produce nanocomposites for biomedical applications.

In conclusion, a new Chitosan-PVP-Nanocellulose composite dressing with symmetrical and asymmetrical structures modified by a thin stearic acid coating has been successfully prepared for application in wound healing. Thanks to the stearic acid coating, we have produced hydrophobic microporous surfaces, while the uncoated side is a macroporous hydrophilic surface. TEM and SEM proved its homogeneity and high porosity.

Symmetrical and asymmetrical Chitosan-Poly(vinylpyrrolidone)-nanocellulose bionanocomposite wound-healing dressings showed almost similar physicochemical properties, such as mechanical properties, high swelling capacity, moderate moisturizing properties and oxygen permeability (the process of coating dressings with stearic acid, seems to be optional, without cytotoxic and antibacterial analyses). The best properties in terms of physiological biocompatibility and antibacterial capacity are produced by asymmetrical dressings containing no more than 3% nanocellulose in the polymer blend Chitosan-Poly(vinylpyrrolidone)-nanocellulose, with stearic acid. The in vivo wound-healing study showed that asymmetric dressings (temporary biological wound-healing agents) with precisely this concentration of nanocellulose biopolymers healed wounds faster than control wounds (without any treatment, and without nanocellulose, or with 5% nanocellulose). However, complete wound closure was expected by day $21^{\text{ème}}$. This can be seen by visual histological analysis (related to histology, the study of the formation of living tissue), in excellent re-epithelialization and dense collagen formation. This bionanocomposite dressing coated by the hydrophobic side of stearic acid, with 3% nanocellulose, could be tried as a wound dressing material, but tested on animals smaller or larger than albino rats, for application to humans (Poonguzhali; 2018).

References :

Poonguzhali, R.; Khaleel Basha, S.; Sugantha Kumari, V.; (2018). Novel asymmetric chitosan/PVP/nanocellulose wound dressing: In vitro and in vivo evaluation. BIOMAC 9127.

New Trends in Conductive Polymer Nanocomposites and Bionanocomposites:

Nanotechnological advances have shed light on the evolution of nanocomposites at the nanoscale. Intrinsic conductive polymers have been widely investigated due to intrinsically mysterious electronic technologies, as well as reduction-oxidation attributes and diverse potential uses in many fields.

With the emergence of nanotechnology, the manufacture of multifunctional conductive polymer nanocomposites (CPNCs) has attracted a great deal of attention in order to improve and multiply their behavior. CPNCs are composed of one or more components, such as graphene, graphite oxide, chalcogenides, graphene nanoplatelets (CNTs), metals, metal oxides, conductive or insulating polymers, biological entities, metal phthalocyanines, porphyrins, and other nanomaterials...

Applications for CPNCs include biological and chemical sensors, electronic nanodevices, electromagnetic interference (EMI) shielding, catalysis and electrocatalysis, energy, microwave absorption, electrorheological (ER) fluids, and biomedicine. The cumulative advantages of CPNCs (conductive polymers nanocomposites) over parent CPs (conductive polymers) have been clearly demonstrated.

Many designs and fabrications of conductive polymer nanomaterials, have emerged, especially CPs in conjunction with materials such as metals, metal oxides, chalcogenides, carbon derivatives, with variable architectural arrangement and oriented multi-component systems. Different synthesis methods result in variable architectural arrangements and nanocomposite dimensions for versatile applications. Thanks to their excellent electronic qualities, CPNCs can be widely explored for use in heart batteries, for example. In addition, they are chemically and biologically high-precision sensors. Conductive polymer nanocomposites protect against electromagnetic waves, corrosion, spark ignition and discharge explosions. When it comes to the design and synthesis of virgin (parent) conductive polymers, the major challenges are to manipulate the inherent electrical conductivity, and to vary the geometric and morphological arrangements of the components, in order to better functionalize these materials. Pure conductive polymers are therefore deficient in terms of throughput and cycle times for biosensors (detectors of complementary DNA, proteins, antigens, antibodies or diseases, also known as biosensors or biochips = medical devices measuring just a few square centimetres). New synthetic routes and alignment procedures capable of facilitating the large-scale manufacture of nanomaterials, based on conductive polymers, need to be provided. Essentially, we should propose methods for characterizing and controlling the crystalline-amorphous architectural distribution of conductive polymers incorporated into nanocomposites (Idumah; 2021).

References :

Idumah, C.I. ; (2021). Review: Novel trends in conductive polymeric nanocomposites, and bionanocomposites. Synthetic Metals, 273 (2021) 116674.

Book summary

You may find this book interesting, dear readers, if you want to be informed about the latest scientific research on the subject of antiseptic bionanocomposites. You'll get the most important general ideas on a subject that captivates the attention of today's passionate medical students.

Book key words :

- Antimicrobial agent.

- Bionanocomposite.

- Biopolymer.

- Metallic nanoparticles.

- Textile Pharmaceuticals.

- Hydrogel.

- Wound healing.

- Anti-inflammatory.

This book has been approved by the following teachers:

- Pr. Mr Zitouni BENABDELGHANI (Thesis Director at the Faculty of Chemistry-USTHB).

- Pr. Mr Mohamed AMARI (Thesis Co-Director at the Faculty of Chemistry-USTHB).

Those said, follow the direction of a thesis, started by Pr. Mehdia GANDI, since 2017, bearing the theme of a research on bionanocomposites, having therapeutic virtues.

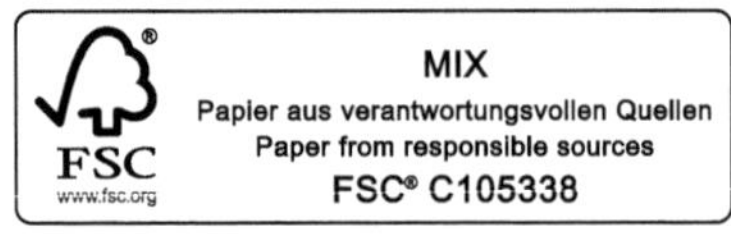

Printed by Books on Demand GmbH, Norderstedt / Germany